THE

HEMOCHROMA

TOSIS

COOKBOOK

SARAH JACK

1

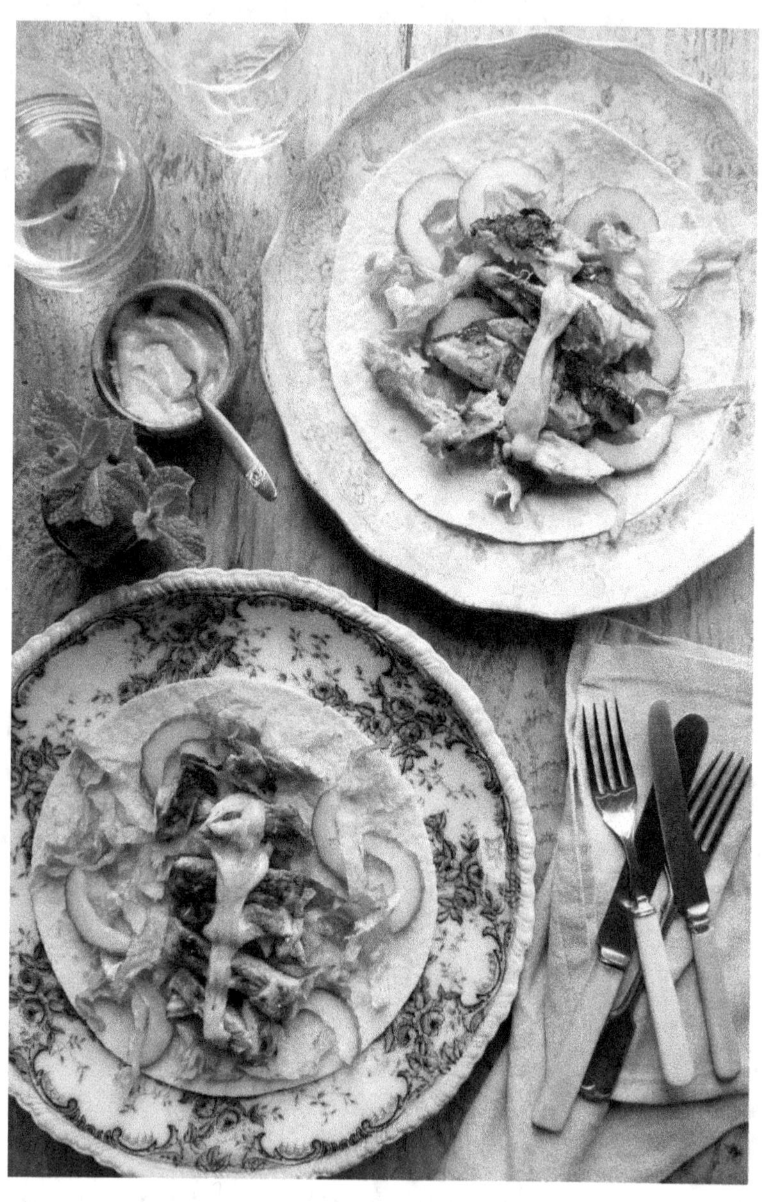

COPYRIGHT

TABLE OF CONTENTS

Table of Contents

INTRODUCTION

HEMOCHROMATOSIS

Hemochromatosis is an inherited condition marked by the excessive absorption and accumulation of iron within the body. Ordinarily, the body regulates its iron levels by absorbing what is necessary and expelling any surplus through liver-produced bile. However, individuals with hemochromatosis experience heightened iron absorption, leading to a gradual buildup of iron in tissues and organs such as the liver, heart, pancreas, joints, and skin.

This surplus iron deposition can inflict harm on these organs over time, resulting in various health issues. Indications of hemochromatosis may encompass fatigue, joint discomfort, abdominal pain, weakness, weight loss, and a bronzed or grayish hue to the skin. Nonetheless, many individuals may not manifest noticeable symptoms until later stages of the illness, when organ damage has already transpired.

The primary cause of hemochromatosis is genetic mutations that disrupt the regulation of iron absorption in the body. The most prevalent form, hereditary hemochromatosis, typically follows an autosomal recessive pattern of inheritance. This implies that two copies of the mutated gene are necessary for its development, one from each parent. However, not all individuals possessing these gene mutations will develop hemochromatosis, as external factors such as diet and lifestyle can also influence the severity of iron accumulation.

Timely diagnosis and intervention are critical in mitigating complications associated with iron overload in hemochromatosis. Treatment generally revolves around the regular removal of excess iron from the body through phlebotomy, commonly known as blood donation. Alternatively, iron chelation therapy may be prescribed to aid in eliminating excess iron from tissues and organs.

Lifestyle adjustments, including abstaining from iron supplements and moderating intake of iron-rich foods and alcohol, may also be recommended to manage iron levels in those with hemochromatosis. Furthermore, genetic testing and screening of family members may be advised to identify those at risk of developing the disorder and implement preventive measures early on.

Overall, while hemochromatosis poses significant health risks if untreated, early detection, proper management, and lifestyle adaptations can enable affected individuals to lead healthy and fulfilling lives. Consistent monitoring of iron levels and adherence to treatment protocols are imperative for upholding optimal health and averting long-term complications stemming from iron overload.

HEMOCHROMATOSIS DIET

Dietary recommendations for individuals grappling with hemochromatosis center on curtailing iron intake to regulate iron levels within the body. Here are some dietary directives tailored to individuals managing hemochromatosis:

Limit Iron-Rich Foods: Minimize or abstain from foods boasting high iron content, such as red meat, organ meats like liver and kidney, shellfish, and iron-fortified cereals and grains. These dietary choices can contribute to excessive iron buildup.

Moderate Vitamin C Intake: Given its role in enhancing iron absorption, individuals with hemochromatosis should moderate their consumption of vitamin C-rich foods and supplements, including citrus fruits, strawberries, and bell peppers, particularly during meals.

Avoid Iron Supplements: Unless expressly recommended by a healthcare provider, steer clear of iron supplements or multivitamins fortified with iron, as they can exacerbate iron overload.

Choose Low-Iron Alternatives: Opt for foods boasting lower iron content, such as poultry, fish, eggs, dairy products, legumes, nuts, seeds, and grains, as these options offer essential nutrients sans significantly elevating iron levels.

Employ Suitable Cooking Methods: Employ cooking techniques that minimize the release of iron from foods, favoring methods like boiling over grilling or frying.

Limit Alcohol Consumption: Given its potential to exacerbate liver damage, restrict or abstain from alcohol consumption to safeguard liver health and mitigate complications linked to iron overload.

Prioritize Hydration: Ensure adequate hydration by consuming ample water, as this can help stave off complications like kidney stones associated with iron overload.

Regular Monitoring: Undergo regular blood tests to monitor iron levels as advised by healthcare professionals. Tailor dietary choices and lifestyle habits based on iron levels to effectively manage iron overload.

Individuals contending with hemochromatosis should collaborate closely with healthcare experts, such as registered dietitians or nutritionists, to devise personalized dietary strategies that align with their unique requirements and medical backgrounds. These professionals offer invaluable guidance on navigating iron intake while safeguarding overall nutrition and well-being. Moreover, genetic counseling and familial screenings may be advocated to identify individuals susceptible to hemochromatosis and implement suitable interventions.

BENEFITS OF HEMOCHROMATOSIS DIET

The dietary recommendations for individuals managing hemochromatosis aim to regulate iron levels within the body, thereby averting excessive iron accumulation and potential health complications. Here are several potential advantages associated with adhering to a hemochromatosis diet:

Iron Overload Prevention: The foremost objective of the hemochromatosis diet is to curtail iron intake from dietary sources, thus thwarting the excessive buildup of iron in bodily tissues. Through avoidance or moderation of iron-rich foods and supplements, individuals with hemochromatosis can help maintain iron levels within normal parameters, diminishing the risk of iron overload.

Symptom Alleviation: Adhering to a hemochromatosis diet may mitigate symptoms linked to iron overload, such as fatigue, joint discomfort, abdominal distress, and skin pigmentation issues. By managing iron levels via dietary adjustments, individuals with hemochromatosis may experience enhancements in overall well-being and quality of life.

Organ Protection: Excessive iron accumulation in organs like the liver, heart, pancreas, and joints can precipitate tissue damage and dysfunction over time. By curbing dietary iron intake, individuals with hemochromatosis can help shield these vital organs from the deleterious effects of iron overload, thereby diminishing the likelihood of complications such as liver cirrhosis, cardiovascular ailments, diabetes, and arthritic conditions.

Optimization of Treatment Efficacy: For those undergoing hemochromatosis treatment modalities like phlebotomy (blood removal) or iron chelation therapy, adhering to a hemochromatosis diet can complement medical interventions by impeding the re-accumulation of iron in the body. Through adherence to a low-iron diet, individuals can bolster the efficacy of treatment, potentially reducing the frequency or intensity of required interventions to manage iron levels effectively.

Promotion of Overall Health: A hemochromatosis diet underscores the consumption of nutrient-rich foods teeming with essential vitamins, minerals, and other beneficial nutrients. By prioritizing a well-rounded and health-conscious dietary regimen, individuals with hemochromatosis can fortify their overall health and vitality, diminish the risk of nutritional deficits, and fortify the body's resilience in grappling with the challenges posed by a chronic condition like hemochromatosis.

Prevention of Complications: Through diligent management of iron levels via dietary adjustments and other lifestyle interventions, individuals with hemochromatosis can attenuate the likelihood of complications arising from iron overload. Such complications may encompass liver maladies, cardiac issues, diabetes mellitus, arthritic conditions, and certain malignancies. Adherence to a hemochromatosis diet can thus mitigate the impact of the condition on long-term health outcomes and enhance prognostic outlooks.

In summary, the merits of a hemochromatosis diet encompass the prevention of iron overload, alleviation of symptoms, safeguarding of vital organs, optimization of treatment synergy, promotion of holistic health, and prevention of associated complications. It is imperative for individuals contending with hemochromatosis to collaborate closely with healthcare professionals, such as registered dietitians or nutritionists, to formulate personalized dietary blueprints

tailored to their unique requisites and health aspirations.

IDENTIFYING LOW-IRON FOODS

Lean Protein Sources:

- ➤ Skinless poultry (chicken, turkey)
- ➤ White fish (cod, haddock, tilapia)
- ➤ Shellfish (shrimp, crab, lobster)
- ➤ Plant-based proteins (tofu, tempeh, legumes)
- ➤ Dairy and Dairy Alternatives:

Low-fat or fat-free milk

- ➤ Yogurt (plain, unsweetened)
- ➤ Cheese (mozzarella, ricotta)
- ➤ Fortified dairy alternatives (almond milk, soy milk)

Grains and Starches:

- ➤ Whole grains (brown rice, quinoa, barley)
- ➤ Pasta (whole wheat, rice, bean-based)
- ➤ Bread (whole grain, sourdough)

> Cereals (low-iron varieties, oatmeal)

Fruits and Vegetables:

> Fresh fruits (apples, berries, citrus)

> Vegetables (leafy greens, broccoli, bell peppers)

> Dried fruits (apricots, figs, raisins)

> Canned or cooked vegetables (without added sauces)

Nuts, Seeds, and Oils:

> Nuts (almonds, cashews, peanuts)

> Seeds (sunflower seeds, pumpkin seeds, chia seeds)

> Nut butters (almond butter, peanut butter)

> Cooking oils (olive oil, avocado oil)

Beverages:

> Water (plain or flavored)

> Herbal teas (chamomile, peppermint, rooibos)

> Coffee (black, with minimal cream or sugar)

➢ Fruit juices (unsweetened, diluted with water)

Condiments and Flavorings:

➢ Vinegar (balsamic, apple cider)

➢ Mustard (Dijon, whole grain)

➢ Herbs and spices (garlic, ginger, turmeric)

➢ Low-sodium sauces and dressings (soy sauce, vinaigrettes)

By incorporating these low-iron foods into your diet, you can effectively manage iron intake and support your overall health, particularly if you have hemochromatosis or need to reduce iron levels for other reasons.

BASICS OF COOKING FOR HEMOCHROMATOSIS

Cooking for hemochromatosis involves careful consideration of ingredients and cooking techniques to manage iron intake effectively. This chapter provides essential guidelines for cooking with hemochromatosis in mind.

Cooking Techniques to Reduce Iron Content:

- Steaming: Steaming vegetables is an excellent way to retain nutrients while minimizing iron content.

- Boiling: Boiling foods can help reduce iron content, especially when discarding cooking water.

- Blanching: Blanching vegetables briefly in boiling water before cooking can help remove excess iron.

- Grilling and Broiling: Cooking methods that involve direct heat, such as grilling and broiling, may lead to higher iron absorption. Use these methods sparingly for hemochromatosis-friendly meals.

➤ Stir-Frying: Stir-frying quickly over high heat can help preserve nutrients while limiting iron absorption.

Choosing the Right Ingredients:

➤ Select lean cuts of meat: Choose lean cuts of meat and remove visible fat to reduce iron intake.

➤ Opt for poultry and fish: Poultry and fish are lower in iron compared to red meat and can be excellent protein sources for individuals with hemochromatosis.

➤ Incorporate plant-based proteins: Legumes, tofu, tempeh, and other plant-based protein sources are naturally low in iron and can be included in hemochromatosis-friendly meals.

➤ Include iron-blocking foods: Foods rich in calcium, such as dairy products, and those high in phytates, such as whole grains and legumes, can help inhibit iron absorption and may be beneficial for individuals with hemochromatosis.

> Avoid iron-fortified foods: Be cautious of consuming iron-fortified cereals, bread, and other processed foods, as they can contribute to excess iron intake.

Flavor Enhancers and Seasonings:

> Incorporate herbs and spices: Use herbs and spices to add flavor to your meals without relying on salt or iron-rich seasonings.

> Experiment with citrus: Citrus fruits and their zest can lend a refreshing acidity to dishes, enhancing flavor without increasing iron content.

> Consider vinegar-based dressings: Vinegar-based dressings and sauces can add tanginess to salads and dishes without adding excess iron.

Meal Preparation Tips:

- ➤ Plan ahead: Plan your meals to include a variety of nutrient-rich, low-iron ingredients.

- ➤ Read labels: Pay attention to food labels to identify products fortified with iron and other additives.

- ➤ Cook in batches: Prepare meals in advance and portion them out for convenient, iron-conscious eating throughout the week.

- ➤ Stay organized: Keep your kitchen well-stocked with hemochromatosis-friendly ingredients and tools to simplify meal preparation.

By adopting these cooking techniques and ingredient choices, individuals with hemochromatosis can enjoy delicious, balanced meals while effectively managing their iron intake and promoting overall health.

HEMOCHROMATOSIS DIET RECIPES

Salmon with Lemon-Dill Sauce

Ingredients:

- 4 salmon fillets

- 2 tablespoons olive oil

- Juice of 1 lemon

- 2 tablespoons chopped fresh dill

- Salt and pepper to taste

Instructions:

- Preheat oven to 375°F (190°C).

- Place salmon fillets on a baking sheet lined with parchment paper.

- Drizzle olive oil and lemon juice over the fillets.

- Sprinkle chopped dill, salt, and pepper evenly.

- Bake for 15-20 minutes or until salmon is cooked through.

Quinoa Salad with Vegetables

Ingredients:

- 1 cup quinoa, rinsed

- 2 cups water or vegetable broth

- 1 cucumber, diced

- 1 bell pepper, diced

- 1/2 cup cherry tomatoes, halved

- 1/4 cup chopped parsley

- Juice of 1 lemon

- 2 tablespoons olive oil

- Salt and pepper to taste

Instructions:

- In a saucepan, bring water or vegetable broth to a boil. Add quinoa, reduce heat, cover, and simmer for 15 minutes or until liquid is absorbed.

- Fluff quinoa with a fork and let it cool.

- In a large bowl, combine cooled quinoa with diced cucumber, bell pepper, cherry tomatoes, and chopped parsley.

- In a small bowl, whisk together lemon juice, olive oil, salt, and pepper.

- Pour dressing over the salad and toss to combine. Serve chilled.

Turkey and Vegetable Stir-Fry

Ingredients:

- 1 lb turkey breast, sliced

- 2 tablespoons olive oil

- 2 garlic cloves, minced

- 1 onion, sliced

- 1 bell pepper, sliced

- 1 cup broccoli florets

- 1 cup snap peas

- 2 tablespoons low-sodium soy sauce

- 1 tablespoon honey

- 1 teaspoon grated ginger

Instructions:

- Heat olive oil in a large skillet over medium-high heat.

- Add minced garlic and sliced onion, cook until softened.

- Add turkey slices and cook until browned.

- Stir in bell pepper, broccoli, and snap peas. Cook for a few minutes until vegetables are tender-crisp.

- In a small bowl, mix soy sauce, honey, and grated ginger. Pour over the turkey and vegetables, toss to coat evenly. Cook for another minute.

- Serve hot over cooked rice or quinoa.

Spinach and Mushroom Omelette

Ingredients:

- 4 eggs

- 1 cup baby spinach

- 1/2 cup sliced mushrooms

- 1/4 cup diced onion

- 1/4 cup shredded cheese (optional)

- Salt and pepper to taste

- 1 tablespoon olive oil

Instructions:

- In a bowl, beat eggs with salt and pepper.

- Heat olive oil in a non-stick skillet over medium heat.

- Add diced onion and sliced mushrooms, cook until softened.

- Add baby spinach to the skillet and cook until wilted.

- Pour beaten eggs over the vegetables in the skillet.

- Sprinkle shredded cheese over the eggs if desired.

- Cook until the edges are set, then carefully flip the omelette and cook until fully set.

- Serve hot with a side salad.

Lentil Soup

Ingredients:

- 1 cup dried lentils, rinsed
- 4 cups vegetable broth
- 1 onion, diced
- 2 carrots, diced
- 2 celery stalks, diced
- 2 garlic cloves, minced
- 1 teaspoon ground cumin
- 1/2 teaspoon smoked paprika
- Salt and pepper to taste
- 2 tablespoons olive oil

Instructions:

- Heat olive oil in a large pot over medium heat.

- Add diced onion, carrots, celery, and minced garlic. Cook until softened.

- Stir in ground cumin and smoked paprika, cook for another minute.

- Add rinsed lentils and vegetable broth to the pot. Bring to a boil, then reduce heat and simmer for 20-25 minutes or until lentils are tender.

- Season with salt and pepper to taste.

- Serve hot, garnished with fresh parsley if desired.

Chicken and Vegetable Skewers

Ingredients:

- 1 lb chicken breast, cut into cubes

- 1 zucchini, sliced

- 1 bell pepper, cut into chunks

- 1 red onion, cut into chunks

- 2 tablespoons olive oil

- 1 tablespoon balsamic vinegar

- 1 teaspoon dried oregano

- Salt and pepper to taste

Instructions:

- In a bowl, combine olive oil, balsamic vinegar, dried oregano, salt, and pepper.

- Add chicken cubes to the bowl and toss to coat evenly. Let marinate for 30 minutes.

- Preheat grill or grill pan over medium-high heat.

- Thread marinated chicken cubes onto skewers alternating with slices of zucchini, bell pepper, and red onion.

- Grill skewers for 8-10 minutes, turning occasionally, until chicken is cooked through and vegetables are tender.

- Serve hot with a side of quinoa or couscous.

Tofu and Vegetable Stir-Fry

Ingredients:

- 1 block firm tofu, cubed

- 2 tablespoons soy sauce

- 1 tablespoon rice vinegar

- 1 tablespoon sesame oil

- 2 garlic cloves, minced

- 1 tablespoon grated ginger

- 1 bell pepper, sliced

- 1 cup snow peas

- 1 carrot, julienned

- 2 green onions, sliced

- Cooked rice for serving

Instructions:

- In a bowl, mix soy sauce, rice vinegar, sesame oil, minced garlic, and grated ginger.

- Add cubed tofu to the bowl and toss to coat. Let marinate for 15-20 minutes.

- Heat a large skillet over medium-high heat. Add marinated tofu and cook until golden brown on all sides.

- Remove tofu from the skillet and set aside.

- In the same skillet, add sliced bell pepper, snow peas, julienned carrot, and sliced green onions. Stir-fry for a few minutes until vegetables are tender-crisp.

- Return cooked tofu to the skillet and toss everything together.

- Serve hot over cooked rice.

Baked Cod with Mediterranean Salsa

Ingredients:

- 4 cod fillets

- 2 tablespoons olive oil

- 2 garlic cloves, minced

- 1 teaspoon dried oregano

- 1/2 teaspoon smoked paprika

- Salt and pepper to taste

For the salsa:

- 1 cup cherry tomatoes, halved

- 1/2 cucumber, diced

- 1/4 cup chopped Kalamata olives

- 2 tablespoons chopped fresh parsley

- Juice of 1 lemon

- 1 tablespoon olive oil

* Salt and pepper to taste

Instructions:

* Preheat oven to 400°F (200°C).

* Place cod fillets on a baking sheet lined with parchment paper.

* In a small bowl, mix olive oil, minced garlic, dried oregano, smoked paprika, salt, and pepper.

* Brush the olive oil mixture over the cod fillets.

* Bake for 15-20 minutes or until cod is opaque and flakes easily with a fork.

* While the cod is baking, prepare the salsa. In a bowl, combine halved cherry tomatoes, diced cucumber, chopped Kalamata olives, chopped parsley, lemon juice, olive oil, salt, and pepper.

* Serve baked cod hot with Mediterranean salsa on top.

Vegetable and Bean Soup

Ingredients:

- 1 tablespoon olive oil

- 1 onion, diced

- 2 carrots, diced

- 2 celery stalks, diced

- 2 garlic cloves, minced

- 4 cups vegetable broth

- 1 can (15 oz) diced tomatoes

- 1 can (15 oz) white beans, drained and rinsed

- 1 teaspoon dried thyme

- Salt and pepper to taste

- 2 cups baby spinach

Instructions:

- Heat olive oil in a large pot over medium heat.

- Add diced onion, carrots, celery, and minced garlic. Cook until softened.

- Pour vegetable broth and diced tomatoes with their juices into the pot. Bring to a boil.

- Stir in white beans and dried thyme. Season with salt and pepper to taste.

- Reduce heat and let simmer for 15-20 minutes.

- Add baby spinach to the soup and cook until wilted.

- Serve hot with crusty bread.

Grilled Vegetable Salad

Ingredients:

- 1 zucchini, sliced lengthwise

- 1 eggplant, sliced

- 1 bell pepper, halved

- 1 red onion, sliced into rounds

- 2 tablespoons olive oil

- Salt and pepper to taste

- 2 tablespoons balsamic vinegar

- 1 tablespoon chopped fresh basil

Instructions:

- Preheat grill or grill pan over medium-high heat.

- Brush sliced vegetables with olive oil and season with salt and pepper.

- Grill vegetables until tender and lightly charred, about 4-5 minutes per side.

- Remove vegetables from the grill and let cool slightly.

- Cut grilled vegetables into bite-sized pieces and transfer to a serving platter.

- Drizzle balsamic vinegar over the grilled vegetables and sprinkle with chopped fresh basil.

- Serve warm or at room temperature.

Cauliflower Rice Stir-Fry

Ingredients:

- 1 head cauliflower, grated into rice-like texture

- 1 tablespoon sesame oil

- 2 garlic cloves, minced

- 1 cup mixed vegetables (such as bell peppers, broccoli, snap peas)

- 2 tablespoons low-sodium soy sauce

- 1 tablespoon rice vinegar

- 2 green onions, sliced

- Salt and pepper to taste

Instructions:

- Heat sesame oil in a large skillet over medium heat.

- Add minced garlic and grated cauliflower rice. Cook for 5-7 minutes until cauliflower is tender.

- Stir in mixed vegetables and cook until tender-crisp.

- In a small bowl, mix soy sauce and rice vinegar. Pour over the cauliflower rice and vegetables, toss to combine.

- Cook for another 2-3 minutes, then sprinkle sliced green onions on top. Serve hot.

Mediterranean Chickpea Salad

Ingredients:

- 1 can (15 oz) chickpeas, drained and rinsed
- 1 cucumber, diced
- 1 bell pepper, diced
- 1/4 cup chopped red onion
- 1/4 cup chopped fresh parsley
- 2 tablespoons olive oil
- Juice of 1 lemon
- 1 teaspoon dried oregano
- Salt and pepper to taste

Instructions:

- In a large bowl, combine chickpeas, diced cucumber, diced bell pepper, chopped red onion, and chopped parsley.

- In a small bowl, whisk together olive oil, lemon juice, dried oregano, salt, and pepper.

- Pour dressing over the salad and toss to coat evenly.

- Refrigerate for at least 30 minutes before serving to allow flavors to meld. Serve chilled.

Turkey and Sweet Potato Chili

Ingredients:

- 1 lb ground turkey

- 1 onion, diced

- 2 garlic cloves, minced

- 2 sweet potatoes, peeled and diced

- 1 can (15 oz) diced tomatoes

- 1 can (15 oz) black beans, drained and rinsed

- 2 cups low-sodium chicken broth

- 1 tablespoon chili powder

- 1 teaspoon ground cumin

- Salt and pepper to taste

Instructions:

- In a large pot, brown ground turkey over medium heat.

- Add diced onion and minced garlic, cook until softened.

- Stir in diced sweet potatoes, diced tomatoes, black beans, chicken broth, chili powder, ground cumin, salt, and pepper.

- Bring to a boil, then reduce heat and let simmer for 20-25 minutes or until sweet potatoes are tender.

- Serve hot, garnished with chopped fresh cilantro if desired.

Greek Yogurt Chicken Skewers

Ingredients:

- 1 lb chicken breast, cut into cubes

- 1 cup plain Greek yogurt

- Juice of 1 lemon

- 2 garlic cloves, minced

- 1 teaspoon dried oregano

- Salt and pepper to taste

- Wooden skewers, soaked in water

Instructions:

- In a bowl, combine Greek yogurt, lemon juice, minced garlic, dried oregano, salt, and pepper.

- Add chicken cubes to the bowl and toss to coat evenly. Let marinate for 30 minutes.

- Preheat grill or grill pan over medium-high heat.

- Thread marinated chicken cubes onto skewers.

- Grill skewers for 8-10 minutes, turning occasionally, until chicken is cooked through.

- Serve hot with a side of tzatziki sauce and pita bread.

Spinach and Feta Stuffed Chicken Breast

Ingredients:

- 4 boneless, skinless chicken breasts

- 2 cups baby spinach

- 1/2 cup crumbled feta cheese

- 2 garlic cloves, minced

- 1 tablespoon olive oil

- Salt and pepper to taste

Instructions:

- Preheat oven to 375°F (190°C).

- Using a sharp knife, cut a pocket into each chicken breast.

- In a skillet, heat olive oil over medium heat. Add minced garlic and cook until fragrant.

- Add baby spinach to the skillet and cook until wilted.

- Remove skillet from heat and stir in crumbled feta cheese.

- Stuff each chicken breast with the spinach and feta mixture.

- Season stuffed chicken breasts with salt and pepper.

- Place stuffed chicken breasts on a baking sheet lined with parchment paper.

- Bake for 25-30 minutes or until chicken is cooked through and juices run clear.

- Serve hot, garnished with fresh chopped parsley if desired.

Vegetable Frittata

Ingredients:

- 8 eggs

- 1/2 cup milk

- 1 tablespoon olive oil

- 1 onion, diced

- 1 bell pepper, diced

- 1 zucchini, diced

- 1 cup cherry tomatoes, halved

- Salt and pepper to taste

- 1/4 cup grated Parmesan cheese

Instructions:

- Preheat oven to 350°F (175°C).

- In a bowl, whisk together eggs, milk, salt, and pepper.

- Heat olive oil in an oven-safe skillet over medium heat. Add diced onion, bell pepper, and zucchini. Cook until softened.

- Spread cooked vegetables evenly in the skillet and pour egg mixture over them.

- Arrange halved cherry tomatoes on top of the egg mixture.

- Sprinkle grated Parmesan cheese over the frittata.

- Transfer the skillet to the preheated oven and bake for 20-25 minutes or until the frittata is set and golden brown.

- Slice and serve hot or at room temperature.

Stuffed Bell Peppers with Quinoa and Black Beans

Ingredients:

- 4 bell peppers, halved and seeded

- 1 cup cooked quinoa

- 1 can (15 oz) black beans, drained and rinsed

- 1 cup corn kernels

- 1/2 cup diced tomatoes

- 1/4 cup chopped fresh cilantro

- 1 teaspoon ground cumin

- 1/2 teaspoon chili powder

- Salt and pepper to taste

- 1/2 cup shredded cheddar cheese (optional)

Instructions:

- Preheat oven to 375°F (190°C).

- In a large bowl, mix together cooked quinoa, black beans, corn kernels, diced tomatoes, chopped fresh cilantro, ground cumin, chili powder, salt, and pepper.

- Stuff each bell pepper half with the quinoa and black bean mixture.

- Place stuffed bell peppers in a baking dish. If using shredded cheddar cheese, sprinkle it on top of the stuffed peppers.

- Cover the baking dish with aluminum foil and bake for 25-30 minutes.

- Remove foil and bake for an additional 10 minutes or until peppers are tender and cheese is melted.

- Serve hot, garnished with additional chopped cilantro if desired.

Tuna and White Bean Salad

Ingredients:

- 2 cans (5 oz each) tuna, drained

- 1 can (15 oz) white beans, drained and rinsed

- 1/2 red onion, finely chopped

- 1/4 cup chopped fresh parsley

- Juice of 1 lemon

- 2 tablespoons olive oil

- Salt and pepper to taste

Instructions:

- In a large bowl, combine drained tuna, white beans, finely chopped red onion, and chopped fresh parsley.

- In a small bowl, whisk together lemon juice, olive oil, salt, and pepper.

- Pour dressing over the tuna and white bean mixture, toss to coat evenly.

- Serve chilled or at room temperature, garnished with additional chopped parsley if desired.

Zucchini Noodles with Pesto Sauce

Ingredients:

- 4 medium zucchini, spiralized into noodles

- 1/2 cup homemade or store-bought pesto sauce

- 1/4 cup grated Parmesan cheese

- Salt and pepper to taste

Instructions:

- Heat a large skillet over medium heat. Add spiralized zucchini noodles and cook for 2-3 minutes until tender-crisp.

- Transfer cooked zucchini noodles to a serving dish.

- Toss zucchini noodles with pesto sauce until evenly coated.

- Sprinkle grated Parmesan cheese over the noodles and season with salt and pepper.

- Serve immediately as a light and flavorful pasta alternative.

Roasted Vegetable Quiche

Ingredients:

- 1 pre-made pie crust (or homemade if preferred)

- 2 cups mixed roasted vegetables (such as bell peppers, zucchini, mushrooms, onions)

- 1 cup shredded Swiss cheese

- 4 eggs

- 1 cup milk or half-and-half

- Salt and pepper to taste

Instructions:

- Preheat oven to 375°F (190°C).

- Place pre-made pie crust in a pie dish and crimp the edges.

- Spread mixed roasted vegetables and shredded Swiss cheese evenly over the bottom of the pie crust.

- In a bowl, whisk together eggs, milk or half-and-half, salt, and pepper.

- Pour egg mixture over the vegetables and cheese in the pie crust.

- Bake quiche in the preheated oven for 35-40 minutes or until set and golden brown on top.

- Let quiche cool for a few minutes before slicing and serving.

Baked Chicken and Vegetable Casserole

Ingredients:

- 4 boneless, skinless chicken breasts

- 2 cups mixed vegetables (such as carrots, broccoli, cauliflower)

- 1 onion, sliced

- 2 garlic cloves, minced

- 1 tablespoon olive oil

- 1/2 cup low-sodium chicken broth

- 1 teaspoon dried thyme

- Salt and pepper to taste

Instructions:

- Preheat oven to 375°F (190°C).

- Season chicken breasts with salt and pepper, then place them in a baking dish.

- In a skillet, heat olive oil over medium heat. Add minced garlic and sliced onion, cook until softened.

- Add mixed vegetables to the skillet and cook for a few minutes.

- Pour chicken broth over the vegetables and stir in dried thyme. Cook for another 5 minutes.

- Pour vegetable mixture over the chicken breasts in the baking dish.

- Cover the baking dish with aluminum foil and bake for 25-30 minutes or until chicken is cooked through and vegetables are tender.

- Serve hot, garnished with chopped fresh parsley if desired.

Shrimp and Avocado Salad

Ingredients:

- 1 lb cooked shrimp, peeled and deveined

- 2 avocados, diced

- 1 cup cherry tomatoes, halved

- 1/4 cup diced red onion

- 1/4 cup chopped fresh cilantro

- Juice of 2 limes

- 2 tablespoons olive oil

- Salt and pepper to taste

Instructions:

- In a large bowl, combine cooked shrimp, diced avocado, halved cherry tomatoes, diced red onion, and chopped fresh cilantro.

- In a small bowl, whisk together lime juice, olive oil, salt, and pepper.

- Pour dressing over the shrimp and avocado mixture, toss to coat evenly.

- Serve chilled as a refreshing and nutritious salad.

Spaghetti Squash with Tomato Basil Sauce

Ingredients:

- 1 medium spaghetti squash

- 2 cups homemade or store-bought tomato basil sauce

- 1/4 cup grated Parmesan cheese

- Fresh basil leaves for garnish

- Salt and pepper to taste

Instructions:

- Preheat oven to 375°F (190°C).

- Cut spaghetti squash in half lengthwise and scoop out the seeds.

- Place spaghetti squash halves cut-side down on a baking sheet lined with parchment paper.

- Bake for 40-50 minutes or until squash is tender.

- Use a fork to scrape the cooked squash into spaghetti-like strands.

- Heat tomato basil sauce in a saucepan over medium heat until warmed through.

- Serve spaghetti squash topped with tomato basil sauce, grated Parmesan cheese, and fresh basil leaves.

Lemon Herb Baked Cod

Ingredients:

- 4 cod fillets

- 2 tablespoons olive oil

- Juice of 1 lemon

- 2 garlic cloves, minced

- 1 tablespoon chopped fresh parsley

- 1 teaspoon dried dill

- Salt and pepper to taste

Instructions:

- Preheat oven to 375°F (190°C).

- Place cod fillets on a baking sheet lined with parchment paper.

- In a small bowl, whisk together olive oil, lemon juice, minced garlic, chopped fresh parsley, dried dill, salt, and pepper.

- Pour the lemon herb mixture over the cod fillets, making sure they are evenly coated.

- Bake for 15-20 minutes or until cod is opaque and flakes easily with a fork.

- Serve hot, garnished with additional chopped parsley if desired.

Turkey and Vegetable Meatballs

Ingredients:

- 1 lb ground turkey

- 1/2 cup grated zucchini

- 1/2 cup grated carrot

- 1/4 cup finely chopped onion

- 2 garlic cloves, minced

- 1/4 cup chopped fresh parsley

- 1/4 cup breadcrumbs

- 1 egg

- 1 teaspoon Italian seasoning

- Salt and pepper to taste

Instructions:

- Preheat oven to 375°F (190°C). Line a baking sheet with parchment paper.

- In a large bowl, combine ground turkey, grated zucchini, grated carrot, minced garlic, chopped onion, chopped parsley, breadcrumbs, egg, Italian seasoning, salt, and pepper.

- Mix until well combined, then shape the mixture into meatballs.

- Place meatballs on the prepared baking sheet.

- Bake for 20-25 minutes or until meatballs are cooked through and lightly browned.

- Serve hot with your favorite sauce or over spaghetti squash for a low-carb option.

Vegetable and Lentil Curry

Ingredients:

- 1 cup dried lentils, rinsed

- 4 cups vegetable broth

- 1 tablespoon olive oil

- 1 onion, diced

- 2 garlic cloves, minced

- 1 tablespoon grated ginger

- 2 tablespoons curry powder

- 1 can (14 oz) coconut milk

- 2 cups mixed vegetables (such as cauliflower, bell pepper, peas)

- Salt and pepper to taste

Instructions:

- In a large pot, heat olive oil over medium heat. Add diced onion, minced garlic, and grated ginger. Cook until softened.

- Stir in curry powder and cook for another minute.

- Add rinsed lentils and vegetable broth to the pot. Bring to a boil, then reduce heat and let simmer for 20-25 minutes or until lentils are tender.

- Stir in coconut milk and mixed vegetables. Cook for another 10-15 minutes until vegetables are tender.

- Season with salt and pepper to taste.

- Serve hot over cooked rice or quinoa.

Mushroom and Spinach Stuffed Bell Peppers

Ingredients:

- 4 bell peppers, halved and seeded

- 2 cups sliced mushrooms

- 2 cups baby spinach

- 1 onion, diced

- 2 garlic cloves, minced

- 1/2 cup grated Parmesan cheese

- 1 tablespoon olive oil

- Salt and pepper to taste

Instructions:

- Preheat oven to 375°F (190°C).

- Heat olive oil in a skillet over medium heat. Add diced onion and minced garlic, cook until softened.

- Add sliced mushrooms to the skillet and cook until they release their moisture and are tender.

- Stir in baby spinach and cook until wilted. Season with salt and pepper.

- Remove skillet from heat and stir in grated Parmesan cheese.

- Arrange bell pepper halves in a baking dish.

- Spoon the mushroom and spinach mixture into each bell pepper half.

- Cover the baking dish with aluminum foil and bake for 25-30 minutes or until peppers are tender.

- Serve hot, garnished with additional grated Parmesan cheese if desired.

THANKS FOR

READING

THIS BOOK.